Meditation
The Beginner's Guide to Serenity

HUGH S. ALLEN

Meditation promotes great well-being, but should be used in conjunction with conventional medical or psychological care — not as a substitute for it. If you are suffering from depression, post-traumatic stress disorder, suicidal thoughts, severe anxiety, or other psychological or emotional distress, talk to your doctor or a mental health professional before practicing meditation.

Copyright © 2015 Hugh S. Allen

All Rights Reserved. No portion of this book may be reproduced by any means without prior written permission of the author.

ISBN: 9798678085115

CONTENTS

1	Introduction	5
2	Benefits of Meditation	10
3	Getting Started	18
4	Basic Postures or Asanas	26
5	Techniques	35
6	The Meditation Lifestyle	50
7	Conclusion	57

THANKS

TO VC FOR SHOWING ME THE PATH TO MINDFULNESS AND FOR BEING GRACIOUS ENOUGH TO ALLOW ME TO MEANDER ALONG IT WITHOUT JUDGEMENT

INTRODUCTION

"There is no need to go to India or anywhere else to find peace. You will find that deep place of silence right in your room, your garden or even your bathtub" – Elisabeth Kubler-Ross

This challenges the myth that meditation is some profound, mystical activity that only the deeply spiritual can engage in or derive benefit from. Although meditation began in the eastern cultures, the quest for enlightenment or self-realization also has a western counterpart.

The famous American psychologist Abraham Maslow, in 1943, developed what is termed the hierarchy of needs, and it is widely accepted to accurately capture the essence of what motivates mankind.

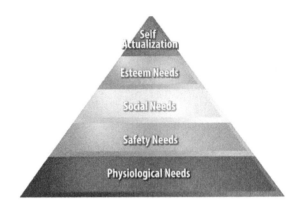

In the hierarchy, Maslow placed 'Self-Actualization' as the highest level of need. This self-actualization represents us at our most content, blissful state because we have reached our highest potential. This directly correlates to the 'Self-Realization' that ancient civilizations have attempted to achieve through meditation for hundreds of years.

To its proponents, meditation is not a technique or practice – it is more appropriately described as a way of life. The word meditation is derived from the Latin words *meditari*, which means 'to think, dwell upon, exercise the mind,' and *mederi* which means 'to heal.' Its Sanskrit (ancient Indian language) derivation *medha* means 'wisdom.' Therefore, meditation can be defined as the practice of bringing awareness to everything you do in order to harness the energy of your mind and body toward expanding and refining your consciousness.

The mind is always full of rambling thoughts; its movements have been likened to that of a monkey constantly jumping from one 'thought' tree to another. At its most basic, Meditation aims to calm our frenzied thoughts and bring our minds to a tranquil, thoughtless state. Through meditation, we typically focus attention on one object, image, or on a singular thought, and as our thought patterns become subdued, it reaches a point where there is nothing left to contemplate; even the object of our focus disappears, leaving the mind completely calm and serene. That state of serenity is considered to be the point of self-realization - where the individual mind becomes one with the cosmic or universal mind.

This is a rather lofty goal for the beginner - the more immediate objective of this book is to guide the reader through meditation to reasonably calm the mind and tap into its power to begin enjoying the many intermediate benefits of meditation.

Once meditation becomes a regular part of your life, you will begin to feel more relaxed, joyful, and totally present in each moment. The regular practice creates a beautiful, self-sustaining dynamic that yields the ever-increasing rewards of joy and peace, which is so addictive that you will want to continue meditating. Over time, as experienced meditation devotees will attest, it will become an indispensable part of your life. Soon you will feel like you are unable to function optimally without your daily meditation. Spending that time, whether it is a lengthy session or only a few minutes, will insulate you with an aura of serenity that will carry you through even the most hectic of days regardless of what may be required of you. It fortifies you, like any nourishing diet would, to face the stresses and wear and tear of modern-day life.

As you develop and become more attuned to your inner resources of joy and peace, you can access them whenever you feel stressed, worried, or afraid. In this book, you will learn more about acquiring that habit of detached observation, which is critical to maintaining an inner poise amidst the chaos. Additional benefits include improved health, greater contentment, better concentration, improved IQ and memory, enriched social interactions, and even the development of creative talents.

This book seeks to discuss these numerous benefits, introduce you to the practice of meditation and provide you with several techniques and tips that will get you started on *and committed to* this remarkable journey. You will find that the discussion has a distinct lean towards tips, a *cheat sheet,* if you will, that will help you to integrate meditation into your life seamlessly and permanently. It is my firm belief that developing a habit of regular meditation is one of the most valuable gifts that you can give to yourself. Therefore, my goal is not only to get you started but to equip you with strategies to make it a regular part of your day-to-day life until it clicks! - then takes on a life all its own.

BENEFITS OF MEDITATION

Meditation is generally considered to be a spiritual practice, but it also has many health benefits. Traditional Western medicine has generally treated the mind and body as separate entities operating independently. Physicians frequently focus on addressing physical symptoms in isolation without considering the complete make-up of the patient. The doctor's office has long been a revolving door where patients enter and leave after the briefest of intervals, prescription in hand, off to try the latest drug developed by the pharmaceutical companies. Only more recently have some health care practitioners been applying a more holistic approach to patient care. This marriage of the sophistication of modern science and a holistic approach to wellness is evident as more health professionals use meditation and yoga techniques to treat and manage life-threatening diseases. Dr. Mehmet Oz, the well-respected cardiothoracic surgeon of The Dr. Oz daytime talk show, practices daily meditation and is a strong advocate of meditation as a healthy practice to adopt. In a video posted on his website in April 2012, he talks about the well-established scientific research that supports its beneficial effects on lowering blood pressure, improving cardiovascular conditions, reducing cholesterol, obesity, and the risk of stroke, among others.

- **Physical.** It leads to a healthy mind and body. With the practice of meditation, the complete human physiology undergoes a change, and every cell in the body is filled with more energy. This results in joy, peace, and enthusiasm as the level of energy in the body increases. On a physical level, meditation:

a. Lowers high blood pressure and improves cardiovascular health by lowering heart rate and improving metabolism

b. Lowers blood lactate levels which reduces anxiety attacks and anxiety levels

c. Decreases tension-related pain like tension headaches, ulcers, insomnia, muscle, and joint problems

d. Increases serotonin production that improves mood and behavior. Low levels of serotonin are associated with depression, obesity, insomnia, and headaches

e. Strengthens the immune system as it receives hormonal messages to curb inflammation as well as increases the production of cells that fight diseases

f. Increases energy levels and teaches the meditator how to channel the inner source of energy

- **Improved Happiness Level.** Meditation leads to a state of calmness and bliss. It can improve relationships and self-esteem. It brings you to a place of clarity, emotional stability, mental alertness, and physical calmness. It increases the production of endorphins long known to create 'feel good' emotions. It also stimulates the parts of the brain that allow us to feel empathy and love while decreasing activity in the parts of the brain that make us feel isolated; it is often given credit for creating a 'natural high.' This is the feeling of bliss that long-time meditators enjoy.

- **Better Stress Management.** Meditation leads to a feeling of calmness and well-being as the heart rate and breathing slow down, and muscles relax, all of which make more oxygen available to the brain. This allows us to be more composed in stressful situations. Meditation can even help resolve the deepest of neuroses, fears, and conflicts that play their part in causing stress and ill-health.

- **Improved Concentration.** Because meditation strengthens the mind, it is able to provide effective guidance to the physical body to successfully execute its tasks. This has been widely used in professional sports, where studies have found a direct correlation between concentration exercises, including meditation, and the performance level of sports professionals. These psychological exercises are a proven way of improving concentration and mental strength.

- **Enhanced Creativity and Intuition.** With regular meditation, the mind becomes very creative and intuitive. It questions established norms and practices that may be considered conventionally logical. In his post on transcendental meditation, Dr. Oz discusses its impact on his own team when he introduced them to meditation. He mentions the "change in the tone and the texture of the dialog away from dwelling on the problems and much more thoughtful, insightful, clever ways of solving problems. Instead of highlighting the issues that were separating us, my team was deriving bliss and joy from finding solutions".

- **Increased Emotional Intelligence.** There is a marked improvement in how one reacts to situations and challenges. One faces challenges with more confidence, the steadiness of purpose, and calmness. You are able to think more clearly, objectively, and deeply. It puts your mind in a state of "relaxed alertness" or mindfulness, which can increase creativity, tranquility, happiness, and optimism.

- **Freedom from Unhealthy Habits.** Meditation can loosen the hold of addictions over your life. Many addictive habits like smoking and drinking can be controlled or completely halted using the practice of meditation. Even food-related disorders like bulimia have been targeted with the practice of meditation.

- **Improved Mental Acuity – IQ Levels and Memory.** While meditation calms some areas of the brain, it stimulates others, including the hippocampus, which converts short-term learning to long-term memory and helps produce more compassion and empathy. It improves attention span, memory, and cognitive function. During meditation, the brain increases the production of dopamine, a hormone that has a positive effect on both memory and information processing.

- **Undisturbed and improved Sleep.** Regular meditation may result in deeper and longer periods of sleep. The practice increases the production of melatonin, which is vital to restful sleep.

- **Improved Social Behavior.** As meditation increases activity in the part of the brain that regulates behavior, it helps control anger, aggression, and compulsive behavior. It leads to a better understanding of life and a more tolerant view, which in turn leads to overall better social interactions.

GETTING STARTED

In the previous chapter, we covered some of the well-documented benefits of meditation. To begin this practice, it is important for you to clarify in your mind what your particular goals are. To clarify, you may ask yourself:

What am I trying to achieve?

How do I want to feel after I meditate?

What are my short and long-term goals?

Once you have a firm grasp of what you are

hoping to achieve, you may formulate your goal into an affirmation that you can easily integrate into your meditation sessions. Affirmations should be expressed in the present tense and in positive language; For example, 'I am confident in social situations' not 'I will not be nervous around people.' For our purposes, it is best to make your affirmation short enough that it can be memorized and recited. This will be your personal statement of intent, so make it a powerful statement that inspires you, and feel free to use it outside of your formal meditation time. Begin your session with your affirmation and use it to close your sessions to reinforce your goal.

In the initial stages, there is no best way to meditate. All methods are effective and powerful, but as you begin to adapt to the practice of meditation, you may gravitate towards a method that you find more suitable for you. At this point, we will not focus on specific postures, although several are discussed later in the text.

As with any worthwhile endeavor, it is

necessary to plan for your meditation. To give yourself the best chance of success, create an environment and sustainable routine that works well for you.

When?

Meditating early in the morning is generally a good time. If you are an early riser, you can get your meditation in before your spouse or kids awake, and you are drawn into the regular routine of family interactions. At that hour, you also have the benefit of the stillness of the morning, which lends itself well to what you are trying to achieve. Also, consider that after a good night's sleep, we tend to wake in a calmer, more tranquil state, with our minds less agitated than it is likely to be as the day wears on.

That being said, it is also important to fit your meditation routine seamlessly into your lifestyle. Your meditation career would be extremely short-lived if you try to wake up at 6 AM to meditate if you have never woken up before 8 AM in your entire life. Find a time that works for you, and then *stick with it!*

Where?

The where of meditating is a profoundly personal decision. I know a stay-at-home mom of young kids who has made her bathroom her personal sanctuary for regular 'spot' meditation sessions whenever literally *she has to go!*

Privacy, of course, is important, so you want to choose a space where you will not be interrupted or distracted by persons entering unexpectedly. Choose a spot that feels peaceful to you. Make sure that you can control any ambient noises, for example, radio and television.

A cluttered area tends to be distracting, as does an area with very bright colors. Neither of these types of spaces will be conducive to quieting your mind.

Think about the things that you love and that are comforting to you. This may be a painting, the smell of a particular flower, or a lit candle. Use the things you love as props in your space to create the sanctuary that will best usher you into a meditative state.

Clothing

Comfort must be your primary concern when you think about clothing for your session. A snugly fitting outfit may be comfortable enough for regular activities but can begin to feel tight and constrictive after you have been sitting still for a few minutes.

Be aware of the temperature in the room and dress accordingly to avoid later distractions if it becomes too cold or warm.

Duration

I often get this question from beginners 'How long should I meditate?' My answer is always the same "Long enough that you end it feeling refreshed but not too long that you feel relieved when it's over." Ten or fifteen minutes is long enough for the beginner to get started with the practice without it becoming a burdensome chore. The key is to gradually increase the time relative to the improvement of your focus and concentration.

Posture

In the next chapter, I will discuss the basic postures that are popularly used for meditation. This section is meant to be a practical start-up guide for the person who may still be intimidated by the traditional poses. The pointers will also help anyone who is unable to do the traditional poses because of physical disability or injury.

For the purpose of meditation, a normal seated position is adequate, or if you are unable to sit up, you can still meditate as long as you can lie on a flat enough surface to keep your spine straight.

- If you will be in a seated position, whether in a chair or cross-legged on the floor, please make sure you are comfortable. Use a cushion for floor seating. Specially made cushions are available online or in specialty shops, but a regular thin cushion will also work well.

- Sit upright, keeping your back straight. It is important to keep the spine relaxed but not slumped. By pushing out your belly slightly and sitting back a bit, it helps to achieve an erect posture without leading to stiffness or causing you to experience discomfort. The proper alignment of the spine is just as important when you are meditating in a supine position.

- Be aware of your neck and shoulders. Although you want to maintain an erect posture, release any rigidity that may be in your neck and un-hunch your shoulders. Allow your arms to relax and hang loosely at your side.

- Relax your facial muscles by focusing on each one. Un-furrow your brows and allow your eyes to close gently. Your mouth and jaw may be tight – unclench your teeth and assume a relaxed expression. Dropping your chin slightly will help you to keep your face relaxed.

- There are several ways that you can place your hand. You may rest your hand comfortably in your lap or place your palms on each knee. You may also place your hands with one nestled into the other, and the tips of your thumbs meeting at the level of your navel. Another option is to place your hands on your knees with palms up and the tips of the thumb and index or middle finger held together in a very traditional meditative stance.

BASIC POSTURES OR ASANAS

Asana means position or bodily posture used for meditative practice. Asana in ancient days was primarily derived from the postures of birds and animals. Of the approximately 800,000 – 900,000 different asanas, only 84 are now known and practiced widely. The most popular of these are discussed here.

Some believe that certain postures generate a different energy or a higher level of efficacy than others. However, it is possible to get the maximum benefit from any pose if done consistently, being careful to adhere to breath control, visual concentration, or the repetition of a mantra. As meditation becomes a regular part of your life, you will find that you have a preference for one or more meditation postures over the others.

LOTUS POSTURE

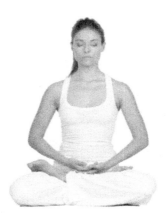

The Lotus pose is the most recognized yoga pose and is the classic pose recommended by many gurus for practicing meditation. Starting from the point of sitting cross-legged, one foot is placed on top of the opposite thigh with its sole facing upward and heel close to the abdomen. The other foot is then lifted up slowly and placed on the opposite thigh in a symmetrical way. The knees are in contact with the ground. The torso is aligned with the spinal column, which supports it with minimal muscular effort.

To a beginner, this position may be difficult and is not recommended if the body is not yet flexible enough to maintain the position *comfortably* for minutes at a time.

HALF-LOTUS POSTURE

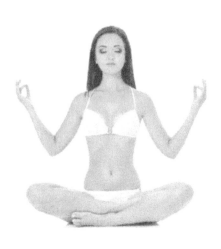

The half-lotus posture is an easier pose than the lotus; however, it may still be challenging for a body that is unaccustomed to this type of movement and positioning. The posture is similar to the full lotus except that one foot is placed on the opposite thigh, and the other foot is resting on the floor. This posture is advocated for those who are not able to go in for the full lotus position. It is traditionally used for long periods of meditation and breathing exercises.

KNEELING POSTURE

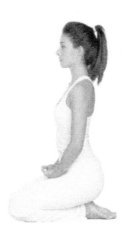

The kneeling meditation posture – also known as Hero pose – is another classic meditation posture. This pose involves sitting on the ankles. You can practice the kneeling pose without any support, but doing so can put considerable pressure on the feet, ankles, and knees. It is much more comfortable to use a meditation cushion or bench. You may also use a stack of folded blankets, or if you're comfortable with only a slight lift, a yoga block will do.

Try to remain upright. Resist the urge to slump by tilting the pelvis slightly forward, so you are positioned on the frontal edge of each sitting bone. Then draw the abdomen back toward the spine to achieve an erect posture.

The hand position that is often used is to interlock the fingers so that they are inside your palms and then extend the forefingers so that they are touching and place the thumbs together.

This posture may be uncomfortable in the beginning but becomes easier with practice.

SITTING CROSS-LEGGED

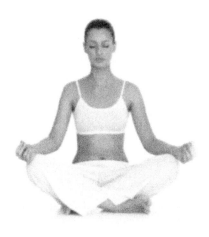

The posture is a simple meditation pose where you sit cross-legged with the feet on the ground rather than on the thighs as in the lotus postures. The feet are placed under the knees with the shins crossed in the center. The knees are level with (or below) the hips. The hands are on the thighs.

Although this is a simple pose to achieve, to enjoy comfort and stability, it may be necessary to use something that elevates you slightly. It may be a meditation cushion, or staples from your linen closet - a folded blanket or a thick towel. You sit towards the front edge of the meditation cushion or blanket and let the hips roll forward slightly. This relieves the pressure on the hip joints, knees, and lower back and allows the legs to relax and fall into place more naturally.

CHAIR POSTURE

Arguably, the easiest of all postures and is strongly recommended for those whose bodies may not be very flexible. It is an excellent jumping-off point for the novice who is just beginning the practice of meditation. Sit comfortably in a chair with your feet on the floor. The spine should be kept erect and should not rest on the back of the chair. Try to lengthen your torso but be careful not to develop tension along the spine due to over-arching in the lower back.

One great benefit of this position is that it allows you to meditate discreetly during your regular activities, such as on a flight or while at your desk at work.

CORPSE POSTURE

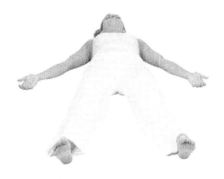

Another very easy posture is to lie like a corpse on your bed or any flat surface with legs spread out and arms resting to the side. For persons with back issues, circulatory problems, or injuries, this may be the only viable posture.

Whether there are physical ailments or not, it is important to be well-aligned, balanced, stable, and comfortable. This may mean using supports like cushions, pillows, or a yoga bolster under the knee. This flattens the lumbar somewhat and puts your back at ease.

Once in a comfortable position, focus your attention completely on your breath, and you may also repeat a mantra to get into the meditative state. This posture can be practiced before going to sleep and is a very popular position for relaxing the mind in preparation for rest. There is a risk of falling asleep, so it is important to remain vigilant to prevent falling asleep prematurely.

TECHNIQUES

BREATH COUNTING

Focusing on the breath is a good starting point in meditation because we can easily find and connect with our breathing. The practice of counting breaths tends to slow down the rhythm of the breathing, settles the mind, and helps to develop concentration. The act of counting also helps to alert us each time the mind has drifted.

It may be instructive to consider the beliefs of the eastern world regarding the importance of breathing in meditation. Hinduism maintains the importance of *prana,* which is the Sanskrit word for 'life force,' or it may also be considered to be absolute energy. Based on Hindu belief, we absorb *prana,* a vital life-sustaining force, each time we breathe in. We rarely think about our breathing - as you inhale and exhale, consider the elementary act of breathing as the valuable life process that it actually is.

You want to mentally count each breath upon exhaling. In the beginning, you may set a goal of a count of ten before re-starting. Keep your attention fixed on the physical sensations of breathing, focus on the tip of your nostrils and upper lip, and observe the air as you breathe in and out. Each out-breath will be a count of 'one' then 'two' and so on until you get to the number ten. Although this is a simple task, it is not necessarily an easy one. You may find that you are continually catching yourself having strayed. Gently bring yourself back to your breath each time with a count of 'one.' At this point, do not be concerned with how many breaths you are able to count before being distracted; the point is to train the mind to quiet itself and achieve focus. Therefore, each time you start back at 'one,' you are being mindful, and that is essential to the training.

MEDITATION: THE BEGINNER'S GUIDE TO SERENITY

As you continue this practice regularly, you will find that your focus becomes sharper. Get more detailed in your observation of your breathing – feel the coolness of the air as you inhale and the warmness of it as it is dispelled. Remain completely relaxed in your face and as the breath naturally slows down and becomes even more subtle, follow it - in and out, in and out, as it traverses your nasal passage.

This method is so useful for calming the mind that it can be helpful as a precursor to another method that you will be using throughout your session, or you can devote the entire session to breath-counting. Simple but profound in its results, this is an excellent tool for the beginner to achieve much sought-after peace and serenity; and it is also important because it ushers you into more advanced meditation practices.

OBJECT-FOCUSED MEDITATION

Using an external object as the focus for your meditation may appeal to you because it has the advantage of allowing you to incorporate something that is meaningful to you directly into your meditation experience. The object may be a personal item, or it may be any other item that you choose. The rule of thumb is to use something that is not too large that it requires you to move your head to see it, but it should be large enough that it doesn't take too much effort to scrutinize. Using an object can be useful because it provides that point of reference that will help you to maintain focus. It is also fairly simple to bring your mind back to the object each time it wanders.

To begin the session, you will want to close your eyes and quiet your mind using some breath counting or just rhythmic breathing. Once your breathing slows down and your thoughts become less agitated, re-open your eyes and focus on your object. Study the object, allowing your mind to observe every detail – its color, shape, texture, and angles. Make sure to use detached observation, therefore do not make any judgments or arrive at conclusions regarding the object. It is merely an item that acts as the center, pulling our usually fragmented thoughts and superficial observations together into a singular focus.

In addition to the peace that one achieves from these object-focused sessions, they open our eyes in a meaningful way to be more observant of our environment. With practice, things that were previously unnoticed will become more vivid and relevant to us. Your appreciation of the 'ordinary' will be enhanced, and thus your experience of life will be enriched.

MANTRA

A mantra is a word or sound that you chant softly as you meditate. The mantra may be a word or phrase that you create from your personal experiences or beliefs. Mantras can be religious or can even take the form of affirmations. You may want to avoid phrases that are too long because the repetition will not have the easy rhythm that is conducive to quieting your mind. The most well-recognized mantra in the western world is the word 'om' which does not have a translation or set meaning but is considered to be a sacred sound that tunes the meditator into the vibration of the universe. Whether you choose to use a prescribed mantra or one that is more personal to you, mantras, when quietly repeated, are very effective at calming a chaotic or easily distracted mind.

To begin, close your eyes and focus on your mantra. Repeat it softly and at an even pace tying it in with the rhythm of your breathing. As with other techniques, the repetition of the mantra will assume a comforting familiarity that can eventually help to usher you into that sweet spot of tranquility very quickly. This becomes especially helpful when you begin to integrate 'spot' meditations into your day.

VISUALIZATION

Visualization has long been considered to be an effective way of creating positive change because of the mind's ability to vividly imagine what one wants to achieve and also because of the

MEDITATION: THE BEGINNER'S GUIDE TO SERENITY

tremendous power of suggestion that it generates. With repetition, visualization is the vehicle that moves you from the imagined state to a shift in your perception of reality. It is this shift that will stimulate new behavior patterns to produce the desired result.

The cocoon imagery is one that is often used. Imagine yourself completely encased in a cocoon that is radiating a bright white light. The light surrounds your entire body until it begins to saturate your being – breathe it in and imagine it permeating every cell of your body, the light glowing through your pores. You are totally bathed in the radiant white light, and it fills you with a feeling of serenity and bliss.

You can remain in this calming, restorative state for the duration of the session, or you can add the dimension of expelling a troubling emotion or problem. It may even be used for healing meditation. While you are surrounded by the cleansing, pure light, you can imagine the problem, addiction, or disease being expelled from your body as black smoke being exhaled through your nostrils or your mouth and losing its potency as it drifts upward and diffuses into the air. You can also envision the negativity as black liquid being forced out by the light and oozing out of your body before being absorbed into the earth without a trace.

A similar concept can be applied using the shrinking box imagery. Imagine a plain, large carton box, open the box, and one by one, begin to place your problems or negative emotions within the box. Once all the objects of negativity are placed in the box, close the box and visualize it becoming smaller and smaller until it eventually disappears.

Visualization as a technique will only be effective with repetition. It will achieve the goal of creating the reality that you desire and rid you of any burdensome problems that you may be experiencing.

WALKING MEDITATION

Combining the act of walking with

meditation may be considered a metaphor for the life we aim to achieve. It is a life lived with greater awareness and mindfulness even as we go about our regular activities and daily interactions. We tend to walk or move from place to place with a destination in mind. Most of us live goal-driven lives that have left us burnt out and stress-ridden. Walking meditation brings our complete attention to the act of walking, we will arrive at our destination, but the destination itself becomes secondary to the journey.

The primary goal in your walking meditation session is to stay mindful at each moment. There is no 'right' way or location or even distance to walk, but it does require some planning to gain as much as possible from the experience. You may consider walking indoors, which offers the best opportunity for you to control your environment in terms of ambient noises, which can become a distraction when outdoors. Of course, walking outdoors in a park or even in your garden if you have a large enough area, can be quite pleasant. Pre-determine the area or distance that you will cover so you will not have to make a decision while walking. For a beginner, it is usually helpful to punctuate your walking area with several required turns; for example, you may walk back and forth on a shorter route or walk along a path that allows you to move as if along the lines of a square. Each time you stop to make that turn, pause and bring your awareness back to the object of your meditation in case your mind has drifted.

You can decide on the best pace for your walk after you have tried it in different ways – each pace has its particular advantage. A slower pace can help to limit distractions; you can keep your lids half-closed without creating anxiety that you may bump into anything. You can coordinate your movements with your breathing which also helps with maintaining focus. At this pace, however, it is possible to get a feeling of being unbalanced as it is not a pace that comes naturally to the body.

A more natural pace can also be used – that would be your regular walking pace. At this pace, you may be less inclined to keep your eyes half-closed, so it gives you a wider angle for your eyes and thus your mind to wander. However, you can counteract that by labeling your steps as you make them to keep your mind focused; try saying "step...step...step" in time with your movements.

Once you have planned your route and are ready to go, take a deep breath and bring awareness to your body – release any tension in your jaw and neck. Your arms should be hanging naturally at your sides, and your legs should feel relaxed. Without focusing on your feet, look downward at an angle of a few feet in front of you. Your gaze should not be fixed but should allow as small a visual cone as possible to avoid distractions. Begin walking and bring your complete attention to your lower legs and feet. Feel your feet as they make contact with the ground, the sensation of your heel touching the ground before rolling the ball of the foot downward. Bring awareness to the contraction of your leg as you lift it, how it feels as it moves through the air and back to placement. If you are walking barefoot, then you will have other sensations associated with each step, the feel of the carpet under your feet, or the coolness of the floor tile. The important thing is to bring mindfulness to the act of walking; because it is such a natural process, the mind is prone to wander; just bring it back gently when you become aware of it.

Some meditators use walking meditation as a natural precursor for their regular meditation because the rhythmic movement helps to focus the mind and sets the stage for a productive session. This is a great way to start your session but engaging in just walking meditation can also yield amazing results. Another advantage of this method is that you can easily incorporate it at other times during your day when you have the opportunity to move from place to place, and this act of mindful walking will continually develop your skills of mindfulness and awareness.

MINDFULNESS AND AWARENESS

These two are more aptly described as attributes of a good meditation session rather than techniques for meditation. They are the over-arching twins that must be present to some degree in your session to make the time that is invested worthwhile. We discussed how agitated and frenetic our natural thought processes can be. It requires some amount of determination and self-discipline to quiet our internal chatter and allow our minds to maintain a singular focus. It is not unusual for completely unrelated and unexpected thoughts to suddenly grab our attention just as we settle into our meditation time. Then we often follow these thoughts down a meandering path for several seconds, maybe even minutes before we catch ourselves off-track. This is not unique to you, so do not be too hard on yourself when it happens. It is important to realize that we are all susceptible to being hijacked by our thoughts and taken away from the present into 'la-la' land at any given moment.

Each time you become aware of drifting, just bring yourself back to the object of your meditation and begin again. With practice, these flagrant wanderings will diminish and may be replaced by other subtler forms of agitation. Remain committed to the process of training your mind, bring mindfulness to each session, and, without judgment, continually bring your mind back to focus, and even the subtler distractions will abate.

In this book, as in other texts on meditation, you will often find references to relaxation and peace, which is likely one reason you are even reading this book. However, it is important to be aware that the word meditation does not connote 'numbness' or 'lack of consciousness.' On the contrary, the meditative state is one of relaxed alertness. There is a mental clarity that should be maintained as we focus on the object of our meditation. In that cocoon of quiet meditation, we have to ensure that we are not overtaken by heaviness and lethargy. This is the reason that novice meditators are cautioned about using the corpse posture because it is quite easy to lose consciousness in such a naturally relaxing pose and cross over into sleep.

The awareness that we bring to each session can help us to keep our meditation charged and sustainable. We have discussed different ways that we can prepare for meditation ranging from our clothing to pre-meditation exercises that can help to set the stage for effective meditation. Awareness anticipates possible distractions and safeguards the mind from wandering away.

Do your best to bring mindfulness and awareness to each session, but it is also important to be patient with your efforts at the outset. If you have ever trained a puppy or even raised a small child, you know that even simple lessons require repetition and reinforcement to be grasped. Your mind is untrained and therefore requires continued practice and time to be able to achieve the calm that will yield the best results. As time progresses, you will find that the peace that you attain in your private meditation carries over into your other activities and interactions. This is when you will truly begin to derive the myriad benefits of meditation.

THE MEDITATION LIFESTYLE

In the previous chapters, we discussed the reasons meditation should become an indispensable part of your life. We looked at the rudiments of meditation, possible postures, and techniques that may appeal to the beginner. This chapter seeks to give you some tips on how to move from being a novice to someone who is enjoying the benefits of meditation in his day-to-day life.

Like any change that you seek to make habitual in your life, meditation will require a commitment. If the benefits that are discussed in Chapter 2 seem appealing to you and you want to appropriate the health, peace, and joy that lie in store – be intentional in your pursuit of this goal. Some simple and very practical tips are listed here to help you to finish strong.

Schedule Your Meditation Time and Block It

Start out by trying some of the more comfortable postures and experimenting to find the technique that most suits you. In the initial stages, it is better to schedule a shorter period of time each day rather than start overly ambitious. Even with a short period, it is important to block it, so it becomes a non-negotiable part of your day. This becomes especially critical on days when you feel discouraged or feel that you are not yet seeing the changes that you anticipate. There are no shortcuts in meditation; it will require practice to start reaping the substantial benefits.

Build on your sessions each day – if you need to re-read specific chapters to help you, do that. It is better to have shorter daily sessions than an hour-long session twice a week. Firstly, it may be more challenging to block two hour-long sessions than, say, a daily ten-minute session; and secondly, you may be setting yourself up for frustration and a higher probability of quitting if you try to start out with such a long session. Make it work for you, keep it easy – use a technique that you enjoy and bring all of your focus into a shorter, more impactful session. Of course, more experienced meditators enjoy lengthy meditation sessions, but they will tell you that it did not start out that way.

Scheduling and sticking with the session routinely may not seem very important at the outset, but it reinforces the idea that this is a lifestyle choice. It also, very importantly, helps to keep you accountable on those days when you want to play hooky.

MAKE IT PERSONAL

In addition to scheduling time to cultivate the practice of meditation in your life and jealously guarding that time, it is also important to make your meditation experience relevant and meaningful to you. In modern life, many of us

MEDITATION: THE BEGINNER'S GUIDE TO SERENITY

experience life as a large crushing ball of activities and tasks that press in on us, continually demanding our attention and jostling for space in our already crowded thoughts. To carve out that time for yourself, establish a routine - a ritual even - that acts as a buffer between you and all the competing tasks and to-do lists. Something as simple as lighting a candle or reciting a well-loved verse from the Bible can usher you into that time of meditation. We discussed earlier the environment in which you meditate - to make it calm and conducive to the peace that you want to channel; Think about those things in your life that are calming; it could be a piece of classical music, a poem, a memorial rock or even a painting. Feel free to incorporate that thing into your meditation time to make it more meaningful to you.

Establishing a ritual that marks the start of your session is an important way of reminding yourself that this is an important time for you. It will help to get you quickly into the frame of mind for meditation, and this will be especially important when you do not have a lot of time, and you want to get the most out of the session, albeit short.

MEDITATION ON THE GO!

Having carved out your regular meditation time, you will become accustomed to thinking about that time of the day as your 'you' time. But what if you could experience more of the same several times throughout your regular day? It could be at your desk at work, in between diaper changes, or even at a red light. Cultivating a habit of taking short meditative pauses throughout the day can be very helpful in maintaining the composure that you achieve in your meditation sessions. Think about it – we spend so many mindless moments during the day when we are paused in traffic, waiting to use the copier at work or in line at the grocery store. There is a veritable treasure trove of time that is available to us that we can spend in quiet focus.

For these quick moments, you will want to relax, bring your consciousness to your body - be aware of hunched shoulders or perhaps a clenched jaw. Breathing exercises are particularly good for these spot meditation sessions; even with only a few available moments, you can take deep breaths, exhale slowly and achieve a deep level of relaxation. Punctuating each day with these brief 'oasis' moments is profoundly satisfying, but the benefit goes way beyond that. Consistent with your desire to establish a meditation lifestyle, you are training your mind each time you do this to shut down the internal chatter to allow you to get to that place of inner peace more quickly and with less effort.

MIND YOUR MOTIVATION

Like the old story about the tortoise and the hare, a slow and steady pace can be more effective than a sprint towards the finish line. If meditation is to become an important part of your life, then allow yourself to enjoy the journey towards that ultimate goal, whatever that may be for you.

As you begin to apply the techniques in this book to quiet your mind, you may be surprised at how frenetic your thoughts are. At the start, it will likely not be easy to stop the barrage of intervening thoughts even when you have created the perfect setting and mood for a productive session. At these times, end each session thankful that for even those brief periods, your focus was intact. Do not become discouraged because you are not seeing the results as quickly as you anticipate. Each successive session builds on the previous and continues the process of training your mind. The value of consistently exercising such a powerful organ should never be underestimated.

When you do not see immediate results, be resolved to continue. You would be hard-pressed to find someone who has invested the time to develop their meditation skills that has regretted it. Be patient with yourself, celebrate small victories, and remember that with the right mindset, the journey can be just as gratifying as the destination itself.

CONCLUSION

It is said that learning to meditate is learning to let go. It is an act of surrender to relinquish the steering wheel and allow ourselves to experience stillness. Our natural inclination is for control – we want to move to the next thing and the next and the next. Our frantic thought patterns lead us to believe that we are adept at multi-tasking because we attempt to juggle all those balls at once. The result is our lives become reminiscent of the hamster busily racing around on his wheel.

Meditation provides us with an opportunity to stop, to quiet our minds, and to create a safe place in which we can truly begin to know ourselves. So, whether you begin your journey seeking healing, stress-relief, or spiritual consciousness, be prepared to let go of the reins and immerse yourself in the stillness. This is the place from which you will emerge energized, enlightened, and empowered. This is your place of peace.

ABOUT THE AUTHOR

Hugh Allen is a self-proclaimed social scientist who has long been fascinated with the mind and its power to effect change. This led him to study eastern healing practices for many years and he is a firm believer in their ability to restore health and wellness.

He has practiced meditation for over fifteen years and leads an informal group of meditation and yoga enthusiasts. In his spare time, Hugh collects vintage music and music paraphernalia and is a regular at local flea markets and estate sales.

ALSO BY HUGH S. ALLEN

- Mindfulness for Beginners

- Pain Management

- Acupressure

Printed in Great Britain
by Amazon